Beginners Guide To Plant Based Diet

Everything You Need To Know About Plant Based Diet Meal Plan To Reset & Energize Your Body With Healthy And Delicious Plant-Based Diet Recipes

Jason Canon

TABLE OF CONTENTS

Introduction

Thank you very much for purchasing this cookbook.

The recipes that I will propose to you are all of vegetable origin, this is to ensure that your body receives all the nutrients it needs.

In this cookbook you will find many recipes to be made with fresh and tasty ingredients, it is a diet based on whole foods of plant origin that will be able to help you lose weight and have a healthier and more balanced diet.

Following a healthy diet is very important for improving your health situation, as well as for losing weight. The recipes in this cookbook are simple but effective and I really hope it's fun for you to recreate them.

Enjoy.

Breakfast Recipes

Tofu Fries

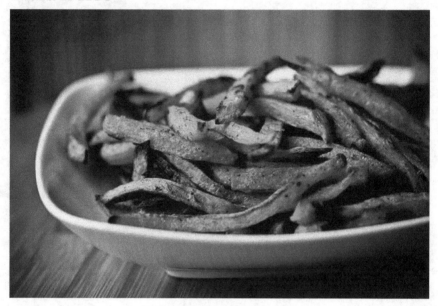

Preparation time: 15 minutes

Cooking time: 20 minutes

Servings: 4

Ingredients:

15 oz firm tofu, drained, pressed, and cut into long strips

¼ tsp garlic powder

¼ tsp onion powder

¼ tsp cayenne pepper

¼ tsp paprika

½ tsp oregano

½ tsp basil

2 tbsp olive oil

Pepper

Salt

Directions:

Warm oven to 375 F. Add all ingredients into the large mixing bowl and toss well. Place marinated tofu strips on a baking tray and bake in a preheated oven for 20 minutes.

Turn tofu strips to the other side and bake for another 20 minutes. Serve and enjoy.

Nutrition: Calories 137, Fat 11.5 g, Carbohydrates 2.3 g, Protein 8.8 g

Chia Raspberry Pudding Shots

Preparation time: 1 hour & 15 minutes

Cooking time: 0 minutes

Servings: 4

Ingredients:

½ cup raspberries

10 drops liquid stevia

1 tbsp unsweetened cocoa powder

¼ cup unsweetened almond milk

½ cup unsweetened coconut milk

¼ cup chia seeds

Directions:

Add all ingredients into the glass jar and stir well to combine. Pour pudding mixture into the shot glasses and place in the refrigerator for 1 hour. Serve chilled and enjoy.

Nutrition: Calories 117, Fat 10 g, Carbohydrates 5.9 g, Protein 2.7 g

Chia-Almond Pudding

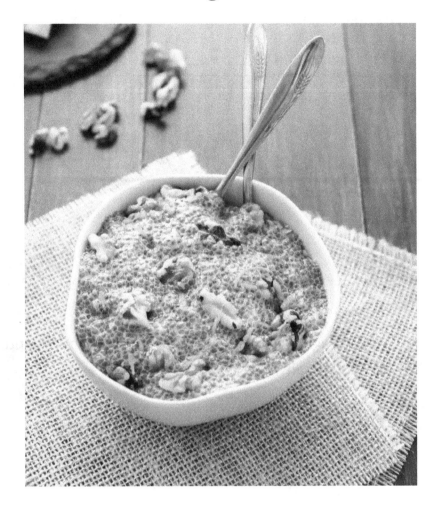

Preparation time: 60 minutes

Cooking time: 0 minutes

Servings: 2

Ingredients:

½ tsp vanilla extract

¼ tsp almond extract

2 tbsp ground almonds

1 ½ cups unsweetened almond milk

¼ cup chia seeds

Directions:

Add chia seeds in almond milk and soak for 1 hour. Add chia seed and almond milk into the blender.

Add remaining ingredients to the blender and blend until smooth and creamy. Serve and enjoy.

Nutrition:

Calories 138

Fat 10.2 g

Carbohydrates 6 g

Protein 5.1 g

Fresh Berries with Cream

Preparation time: 15 minutes

Cooking time: 0 minutes

Servings: 1

Ingredients:

1/2 cup coconut cream

1 oz strawberries

1 oz raspberries

1/4 tsp vanilla extract

Directions:

Add all fixings into the blender and blend until smooth. Pour in serving bowl and top with fresh berries. Serve and enjoy.

Nutrition:Calories 303, Fat 28.9 g, Carbohydrates 12 g, Protein 3.3 g

Lunch Recipes

VEGAN Macaroni and Cheese

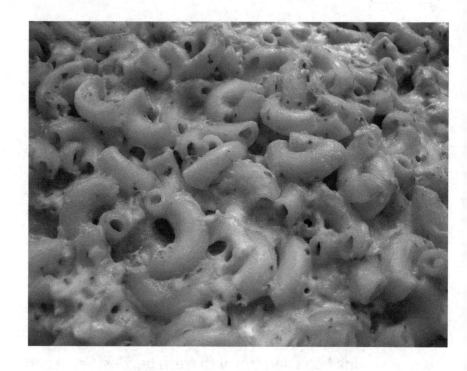

Preparation Time: 15 minutes

Cooking Time: 20 minutes

Servings: 4

Ingredients:

Elbow macaroni, whole grain, eight ounces, cooked

Nutritional yeast, one quarter cup

Garlic, minced, two tablespoons

Apple cider vinegar, two teaspoons

Broccoli, one head with florets cut into bite-sized pieces

Water, one cup (more if needed)

Garlic powder, one half teaspoon

Avocado oil, two tablespoons

Red pepper, flakes, one eighth teaspoon

Onion, yellow, chopped, one cup

Salt, one half teaspoon

Russet potato, peeled and grated, one cup (about two small potatoes)

Dry mustard powder, one half teaspoon

Onion powder, one half teaspoon

Directions:

Cook the broccoli for five minutes in boiling water. Add the cooked broccoli to the cooked pasta in a large mixing bowl.

Cook the onion in the avocado oil for five minutes, then stir in the red pepper flakes, garlic, salt, mustard powder, garlic powder, grated potato, and onion powder. Cook this for three minutes and then pour in the water and mix well. Cook this for eight to ten minutes or until the potatoes are soft.

Pour all of this mixture carefully into a blender and add in the nutritional yeast and the vinegar and then blend. When this is creamy and smooth, then pour it into the mixing bowl and mix well with the broccoli and pasta.

Nutrition: calories 506 fat 22 carbs 67 protein 18

Cilantro Lime Coleslaw

Preparation Time: 5 minutes

Cooking Time: 0 minutes

Servings: 5

Ingredients:

Avocados, two

Garlic, minced, one tablespoon

Coleslaw, ready-made in a bag, fourteen ounces

Cilantro, fresh leaves, one-quarter cup minced

Salt, one half teaspoon

Lime juice, two tablespoons

Water, one quarter cup

Directions:

Except for the slaw mix, put all of the ingredients that are listed into a blender. Blend these ingredients well until they are creamy and smooth.

Mix the coleslaw mix in with this dressing and then toss it gently to mix it well.

Keep the mixed coleslaw in the refrigerator until you are ready to serve.

Nutrition: calories 119 fat 3 carbs 3 protein 3

Delicious Broccoli

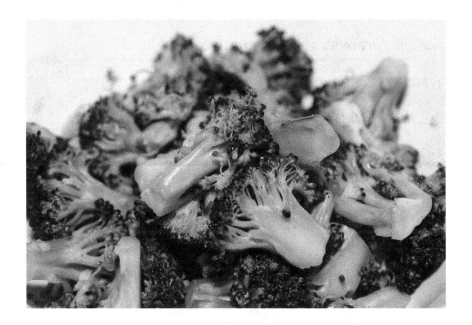

Preparation Time: 15 minutes

Cooking Time: 15 minutes

Servings: 8

Ingredients:

2 oranges, sliced in half

1 lb. broccoli rabe

2 tablespoons sesame oil, toasted

Salt and pepper to taste

1 tablespoon sesame seeds, toasted

Directions:

Pour the oil into a pan over medium heat.

Add the oranges and cook until caramelized.

Transfer to a plate.

Put the broccoli in the pan and cook for 8 minutes.

Squeeze the oranges to release juice in a bowl.

Stir in the oil, salt, and pepper.

Coat the broccoli rabe with the mixture.

Sprinkle seeds on top.

Nutrition: calories 432 fat 1 carbs 24 protein 12

Spicy Peanut Soba Noodles

Preparation Time: 7 minutes

Cooking Time: 17 minutes

Servings: 1

Ingredients:

5 ounces uncooked soba noodles

½ tablespoon low sodium soy sauce

1 clove garlic, minced

4 teaspoons water

1 small head broccoli, cut into florets

½ cup carrot

¼ cup finely chopped scallions

3 tablespoons peanut butter

1 tablespoon honey

1 teaspoon crushed red pepper flakes

2 teaspoons vegetable oil

4 ounces button mushrooms, discard stems

3 tablespoons peanuts, dry roasted, unsalted

Directions:

Cook soba noodles following the directions on the package.

Add peanut butter, honey, water, soy sauce, garlic, and red pepper flakes. Whisk until well combined.

Place a skillet over medium heat. Add oil. When the oil is heated, add broccoli and sauté for a few minutes until crisp as well as tender.

Add mushrooms and sauté until the mushrooms are tender. Turn off the heat.

Add the sauce mixture and carrots and mix well.

Crush the peanuts by rolling with a rolling pin.

Divide the noodles into bowls. Pour sauce mixture over it. Sprinkle scallions and peanuts on top and serve.

Nutrition: calories 512 fat 11 carbs 20 protein 8

Dinner Recipes

Coconut Avocado

Preparation Time: 10 minutes

Cooking Time: 0 minutes

Servings: 2

Ingredients:

2 avocados, halved, pitted and roughly cubed

1 teaspoon dried thyme

2 tablespoons coconut cream

1 cup spring onions, chopped

1 teaspoon turmeric powder

Salt and black pepper to the taste

¼ teaspoon cayenne pepper

½ teaspoon onion powder

½ teaspoon garlic powder

1 teaspoon paprika

Salt and black pepper to the taste

2 tablespoons lemon juice

Directions:

In a bowl, mix the avocados with the thyme, coconut cream and the other ingredients, toss, divide between plates and serve.

Nutrition:

calories 160

fat 6.9

fiber 7

carbs 12

protein 7

Avocado Cream

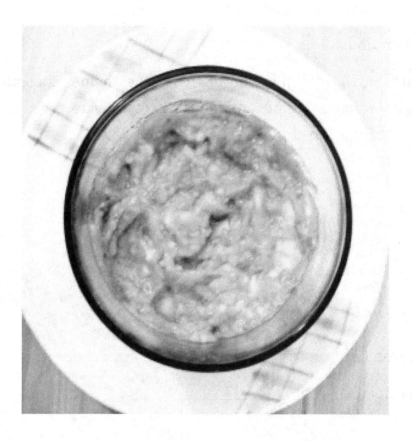

Preparation Time: 10 minutes

Cooking Time: 0 minutes

Servings: 4

Ingredients:

2 avocados, pitted, peeled and chopped

3 cups veggie stock

1 teaspoon curry powder

1 teaspoon cumin, ground

1 teaspoon basil, dried

2 scallions, chopped

Salt and black pepper to the taste

2 tablespoons coconut oil

2/3 cup coconut cream, unsweetened

Directions:

In a blender, mix the avocados with the stock, curry powder and the other ingredients, blend and serve.

Nutrition:

calories 212

fat 8

fiber 4

carbs 6.1

protein 4.1

Tamarind Avocado Bowls

Preparation Time: 10 minutes

Cooking Time: 0 minutes

Servings: 2

Ingredients:

1 teaspoon cumin seeds

1 tablespoon olive oil

½ teaspoon garam masala

1 teaspoon ground ginger

2 avocados, peeled, pitted and roughly cubed

1 mango, peeled, and cubed

1 cup cherry tomatoes, halved

½ teaspoon cayenne pepper

1 teaspoon turmeric powder

3 tablespoons tamarind paste

Directions:

In a bowl, mix the avocados with the mango and the other ingredients, toss and serve.

Nutrition:

calories 170

fat 4.5

fiber 3

carbs 5

protein 6

Onion and Tomato Bowls

Preparation Time: 10 minutes

Cooking Time: 0 minutes

Servings: 4

Ingredients:

1 tablespoon olive oil

2 red bell peppers, cut into thin strips

2 red onions, cut into thin strips

Salt and black pepper to the taste

1 teaspoon dried basil

1-pound tomatoes, cut into wedges

1 teaspoon balsamic vinegar

1 teaspoon sweet paprika

Directions:

In a bowl, mix the peppers with the onions and the other ingredients, toss and serve.

Nutrition:

calories 107

fat 4.5

fiber 2

carbs 7.1

protein 6

Vegetables Recipes

Spicy Swiss Chard

Preparation Time: 10 minutes

Cooking Time: 10 minutes

Serving: 4

Ingredient:

2 tablespoons olive oil

1 onion, chopped

2 bunches Swiss chard

3 garlic cloves, minced

½ teaspoon red pepper flakes (or to taste)

Juice of ½ lemon

Direction

In a big pot, cook olive oil over medium-high heat until it shimmers. Cook the onion and chard stems for 5 minutes.

Cook chard leaves for 1 minute. Stir in the garlic and pepper flakes. Cover and cook for 5 minutes. Stir in the lemon juice. Season with salt and serve immediately.

Nutrition:

94 Calories

5g Fiber

7g Protein

Red Peppers and Kale

Preparation Time: 5 minutes

Cooking Time: 15 minutes

Serving: 4

Ingredient:

2 bunches kale

3 tablespoons olive oil

½ onion, chopped

2 red bell peppers, cut into strips

3 garlic cloves, minced

¼ teaspoon red pepper flakes

Direction

1. In steamer basket in a pan, steam the kale until it softens, 5 to 10 minutes. Remove from the heat and set aside.

2. Meanwhile, in a sauté pan, heat the olive oil over medium-high heat until it -shimmers. Cook onion and bell peppers for 5 minutes. Cook garlic for 30 seconds. Take out from heat and stir in the kale and red pepper flakes. Season and serve immediately.

Nutrition:

101 Calories

5g Fiber

10g Protein

Mashed Cauliflower with Roasted Garlic

Preparation Time: 5 minutes

Cooking Time: 10 minutes

Serving: 4

Ingredient:

2 heads cauliflower, cut into small florets

1 tablespoon olive oil

8 jarred roasted garlic cloves

2 teaspoons chopped fresh rosemary

Sea salt

Freshly ground black pepper

1 tablespoon chopped fresh chives

Direction

Boil cauliflower florets for 9 minutes, then drain.

In a blender or food processor, combine the cauliflower, olive oil, garlic, and -rosemary and process until smooth. Season with salt and pepper. Stir in the chives and serve hot.

Nutrition:

88 Calories

1g Fiber

2g Protein

Steamed Broccoli with Walnut Pesto

Preparation Time: 5 minutes

Cooking Time: 10 minutes

Serving: 4

Ingredient:

1-pound broccoli florets

2 cups chopped fresh basil

¼ cup olive oil

4 garlic cloves

½ cup walnuts

Pinch of cayenne pepper

Direction:

1. Put the broccoli in a large pot and cover with water. Bring to a simmer over medium-high heat and cook until the broccoli is tender, about 5 minutes.

2. Process basil, olive oil, garlic, walnuts, and cayenne for ten 1-second pulses, scraping down the bowl halfway through processing.

3. Drain and put again to the pan. Toss with the pesto. Serve immediately.

Nutrition:

101 Calories

3g Fiber

5g Protein

Finger Food

Pineapple Coconut Detox Smoothie

Preparation time: 10 minutes

Cooking time: 0 minutes

Servings: 2

Ingredients:

4 cups kale, chopped

2 cups of coconut water

2 bananas

2 cups pineapple

Directions:

Add all the listed Ingredients: to a blender

Blend until you have a smooth and creamy texture

Serve chilled and enjoy!

Nutrition: Calories: 299 , Fat: 1.1g , Carbohydrates: 71.5g, Protein: 7.9g

Avocado Detox Smoothie

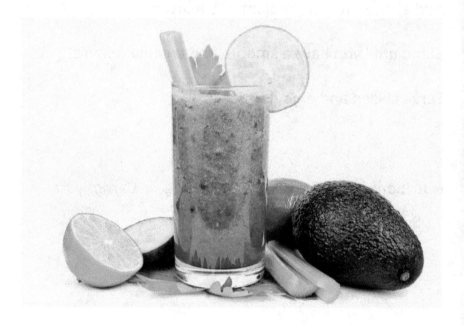

Preparation time: 10 minutes

Cooking time: 0 minutes

Servings: 3

Ingredients:

4 cups spinach, chopped

1 avocado, chopped

3 cups apple juice

2 apples, unpeeled, cored and chopped

Directions:

Add all the listed Ingredients: to a blender

Blend until you have a smooth and creamy texture

Serve chilled and enjoy!

Nutrition:

Calories: 336

Fat: 13.8g

Carbohydrates: 55.8g

Protein: 3g

Lemon Lime Lavender Smoothie

Preparation time: 10 minutes

Cooking time: 0 minutes

Servings: 3

Ingredients:

1½ cups of plant yogurt

3 tablespoons of lemon juice

4 tablespoons of lime juice

A drop of lavender extract, culinary or ½ teaspoon of culinary lavender buds

¼ cup of ice

½ teaspoon of turmeric (or even more to accomplish the desired color)

¼ cup of shavings from fresh organic lemons and limes

Directions:

Combine all of the ingredients in a blender and serve chilled with citrus shavings and lavender buds at the top for a robust scent while you spoon!

Then add plant-based milk to a thin mixture.

Nutrition:

Calories: 229

Fat: 1.1g

Carbohydrates: 71.5g

Protein: 7.9g

Jalapeno Lime and Mango Protein Smoothie

Preparation time: 10 minutes

Cooking time: 0 minutes

Servings: 2

Ingredients:

A little banana

1 Cheribundi Tart Cherry Mango smoothie pack (or ¾ cup frozen mango)

A heaping tablespoon of chopped jalapeño (about ½ a little pepper)

1 cup unsweetened original almond milk (or coconut milk)

1 tablespoon flaxseed, ground

1 tablespoon chia seeds, ground

2 tablespoons hemp seed, ground

½ lime, newly squeezed

½ an avocado (optional)

Directions:

Combine all of the ingredients within a blender and work for approximately 45 seconds until smooth.

Pour right into a glass and revel in!

Nutrition:

Calories: 219

Fat: 1.1g

Carbohydrates: 1.5g

Protein: 7.9g

Cinnamon Apple Smoothie

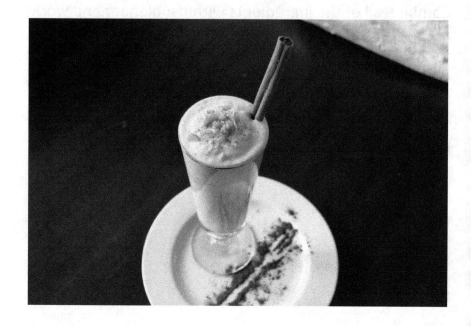

Preparation time: 10 minutes

Cooking time: 0 minutes

Servings: 2

Ingredients:

1 small apple, sliced

½ cup of rolled oats

½ teaspoon of cinnamon

½ teaspoon of nutmeg

1 tablespoon almond butter

½ cup of unsweetened coconut milk three to four ice

½ cup of cool water

Directions:

Combine oats and water inside a blender and allow it to rest for two minutes; therefore, the oats can soften.

Bring all of the remaining ingredients to the blender and blend for approximately 30 seconds until smooth.

Pour right into a glass and sprinkle with just a little spare cinnamon and nutmeg. Enjoy!

Nutrition:

Calories: 232

Fat: 1.1g

Carbohydrates: 14.5g

Protein: 7.9g

Infused Water

Preparation time: 5 minutes

Cooking time: 20 minutes

Servings: 12

Ingredients:

1 lemon

1 orange

1 tablespoon fresh ginger

5 cardamom pods

1/4 teaspoon peppercorn

1 cinnamon stick

6 cups water

Directions:

Cut orange and lemon into slices and smash the cardamom pods. Peel the ginger and slice it up.

Add all Ingredients: to a pot and bring to a boil. Once boiling, stir and reduce the heat to a simmer. Let it simmer until the fruit slices break down.

Strain the liquid into a glass and serve with sugar if desired.

Nutrition:

Calories 17

Sodium 4 mg

Total Carbs 4.3 g

Fiber 1.3 g

Sugar 1.6 g

Protein 0.5 g

Potassium 68 mg

Elixirs

Preparation time: 10 minutes

Cooking time: 0 minutes

Servings: 2

Ingredients:

Nutrition:

Calories: 149

Protein: 3 Grams

Fat: 3 Grams

Carbs: 29 Grams

1 Cup Riced Cauliflower, Frozen

1 Cup Banana, Sliced & Frozen

1/2 Cup Mixed Berries, Frozen

2 Cups Almond Milk, Unsweetened

2 Teaspoons Maple syrup, Pure & Optional

Directions:

Blend until mixed well

Interesting Facts: This vegetable is an extremely high source of vitamin A, vitamin B1, B2 and B3. It has even been said that it can be used as a stress reliever!

Iced Teas

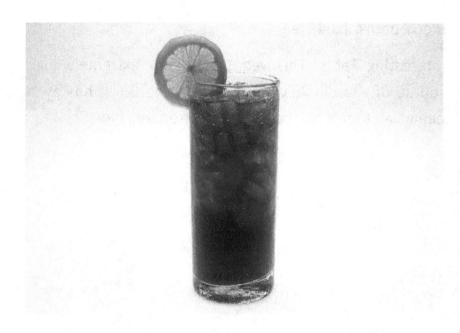

Preparation time: 5 minutes

Cooking time: 0 minutes

Servings: 2

Ingredients:

A cup high quality tea bag

A tablespoon of coconut butter

A tablespoon of plant-based milk of your choice

Optional add-ins:

1 teaspoon of MCT oil

1 teaspoon of cinnamon

1 teaspoon of vanilla powder

1 teaspoon of coconut milk powder (instead of the plant milk)

Directions:

Brew your coffee – either a French press or automatic coffee maker using high-quality coffee.

Add a cup of coffee in a blender along with coconut butter and other add-ins and blend until foamy.

Pour in a mug and top with foamed plant milk or dust with cinnamon.

Nutrition: Calories 73 , Total Fat 2.2 g , Cholesterol 1 mg , Sodium 9 mg , Total Carbs 11.7 g , Fiber 1.6 g , Sugar 6.2 g , Protein2.3 g

Latte

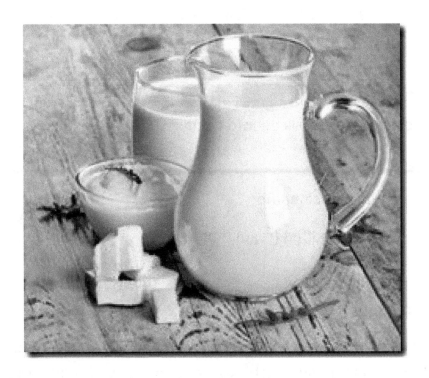

Preparation time: 5 minutes

Cooking time: 0 minutes

Servings: 2

Ingredients:

1/4 cup almond or non-dairy milk

2 tablespoon hemp seeds

Splash vanilla extract

Frozen bananas, sliced into coins

Handful of ice

A few pinches cinnamon

1 cup cooled coffee (regular or decaf)

Directions:

Add the ice and keep blending on high until there are no lumps remaining. Taste for sweetness and add your preferred plant-based sugar or sugar alternative.

Transfer to a glass and serve.

Nutrition: Calories 73 , Total Fat 2.2 g , Sodium 9 mg , Total Carbs 11.7 g , Fiber 1.6 g , Sugar 6.2 g , Protein2.3 g

Soup and Stew

Coconut and Grilled Vegetable Soup

Preparation Time: 10 Minutes

Cooking Time: 45 Minutes

Servings: 4

Ingredients:

2 small red onions cut into wedges

2 garlic cloves

10 oz. butternut squash, peeled and chopped

10 oz. pumpkins, peeled and chopped

4 tbsp melted vegan butter

Salt and black pepper to taste

1 cup of water

1 cup unsweetened coconut milk

1 lime juiced

¾ cup vegan mayonnaise

Toasted pumpkin seeds for garnishing

Directions:

Preheat the oven to 400 F.

On a baking sheet, spread the onions, garlic, butternut squash, and pumpkins and drizzle half of the butter on top. Season with salt, black pepper, and rub the seasoning well onto the vegetables. Roast in the oven for 45 minutes or until the vegetables are golden brown and softened.

Transfer the vegetables to a pot; add the remaining ingredients except for the pumpkin seeds and using an immersion blender puree the ingredients until smooth.

Dish the soup, garnish with the pumpkin seeds and serve warm.

Nutrition:

Calories 290

Fat 10 g

Protein 30 g

Carbohydrates 0 g

Celery Dill Soup

Preparation Time: 5 Minutes

Cooking Time: 25 Minutes

Servings: 4

Ingredients:

2 tbsp coconut oil

½ lb. celery root, trimmed

1 garlic clove

1 medium white onion

¼ cup fresh dill, roughly chopped

1 tsp cumin powder

¼ tsp nutmeg powder

1 small head cauliflower, cut into florets

3½ cups seasoned vegetable stock

5 oz. vegan butter

Juice from 1 lemon

¼ cup coconut cream

Salt and black pepper to taste

Directions:

Melt the coconut oil in a large pot and sauté the celery root, garlic, and onion until softened and fragrant, 5 minutes.

Stir in the dill, cumin, and nutmeg, and stir-fry for 1 minute. Mix in the cauliflower and vegetable stock. Allow the soup to boil for 15 minutes and turn the heat off.

Add the vegan butter and lemon juice, and puree the soup using an immersion blender.

Stir in the coconut cream, salt, black pepper, and dish the soup.

Serve warm.

Nutrition:

Calories 320

Fat 10 g

Protein 20 g

Carbohydrates 30 g

Broccoli Fennel Soup

Preparation Time: 15 Minutes

Cooking Time: 10 Minutes

Servings: 4

Ingredients:

1 fennel bulb, white and green parts coarsely chopped

10 oz. broccoli, cut into florets

3 cups vegetable stock

Salt and freshly ground black pepper

1 garlic clove

1 cup dairy-free cream cheese

3 oz. vegan butter

½ cup chopped fresh oregano

Directions:

In a medium pot, combine the fennel, broccoli, vegetable stock, salt, and black pepper. Bring to a boil until the vegetables soften, 10 to 15 minutes.

Stir in the remaining ingredients and simmer the soup for 3 to 5 minutes.

Adjust the taste with salt and black pepper, and dish the soup.

Serve warm.

Nutrition:

Calories 240

Fat 0 g

Protein 0 g

Carbohydrates 20 g

Appetizer

Easy Stovetop Bread

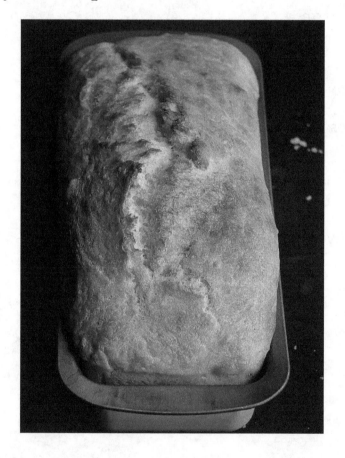

Preparation Time: 15 minutes

Cooking Time: 10 minutes

Servings: 4

Ingredients:

1 cup all-purpose flour

1 teaspoon baking powder

2 tablespoons olive oil

½ teaspoon salt

1/3 cup warm water

½ teaspoon rosemary

½ teaspoon herbs of choice

Directions:

Combine flour, baking powder, plus salt in a mixing bowl. Stir in olive oil and water. Stir until combined, but do not over-process.

Oiled a skillet with olive oil then warm over medium heat. Shape the dough into 4 patties. Drop the dough into the skillet. Cook each side for 5 minutes.

Sprinkle herbs on each side while cooking. Serve immediately or microwave when ready to consume.

Nutrition: Calories 165, Fat 8 g, Protein 4 g, Carbs 23 g

Oven Potato Fries

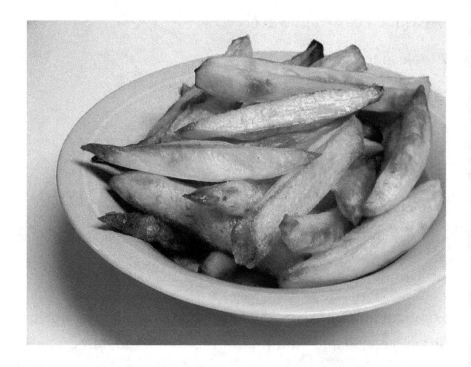

Preparation Time: 15 minutes

Cooking Time: 30 minutes

Servings: 1

Ingredients:

2 ½ pounds Baking potatoes

1 tsp Vegetable oil

1 tbsp White sugar

1 tsp Salt

1 pinch Ground cayenne pepper

Directions:

Start by preheating the oven by setting the temperature to 450 degrees Fahrenheit. Take a baking sheet and line it with a foil. Spray the sheet with a generous amount of cooking spray.

Scrub well to clean the potatoes. Cut each potato into half an inch-thick strips.

Take a large-sized mixing bowl and toss in the potato strips. Add in the vegetable oil, salt, cayenne pepper and sugar.

Place the coated fries on the baking tray lined with cooking spray. Place the baking sheet in the preheated oven and bake for about 30 minutes. Transfer onto a serving platter and serve right away.

Nutrition:

Calories: 263

Carbs: 35g

Fat: 12g

Protein: 4g

Mushrooms with Herbs and White Wine

Preparation Time: 10 minutes

Cooking Time: 15 minutes

Servings: 1

Ingredients

1 tbsp Olive oil

1 ½ pound Fresh mushrooms

1 tsp Italian seasoning

¼ cup Dry white wine

2 cloves Garlic (minced)

Salt, as per taste

Pepper, as per taste

2 tbsp Fresh chives (chopped)

Directions:

Start by heating the olive oil by placing the nonstick skillet on medium-high flame. Once the oil is heated, toss in the mushrooms. Sprinkle the Italian seasoning and sauté for about 10 minutes. Keep stirring.

Pour in the dry white wine and toss in the garlic. Continue to cook for about 3-4 minutes. Season with pepper and salt. Sprinkle the chives and cook for about a minute. Move into a serving bowl then serve hot.

Nutrition:

Calories: 522

Carbs: 27g

Fat: 16g

Protein: 55g

Zucchini Stuffed with Mushrooms and Chickpeas

Preparation Time: 30 minutes

Cooking Time: 30 minutes

Servings: 1

Ingredients:

4 zucchinis (halved)

1 tbsp olive oil

1 onion (chopped)

2 cloves garlic (crushed)

½ package button mushrooms, sliced (8 ounces)

1 tsp ground coriander

1 ½ tsp ground cumin

1 can chickpeas (15.5 ounce)

½ lemon (juiced)

2 tbsp fresh parsley (chopped)

sea salt, as per taste

ground black pepper, as per taste

Directions:

Start by preheating the oven by setting the temperature to 350 degrees Fahrenheit. Take a shallow nonstick baking dish and grease it generously.

Use a spoon to scoop out the flesh in the center of zucchini halves. Chop the flesh into Place the zucchini halves onto the greased baking dish.

In the meanwhile, take a large nonstick skillet and place it over medium flame. Toss in the onions and sauté for about 5 minutes. Add in the garlic and sauté for 2 more minutes.

Now add in the mushrooms and zucchini. Keep stirring and cook for about 5 minutes.

Add in the chickpeas, cumin, coriander, parsley, lemon juice, pepper and salt. Mix well to combine.

Put the zucchini shells on your baking sheet and fill with the chickpea mixture. Put the baking sheet in your oven and bake for about 40 minutes.

Once done, remove from the oven and transfer onto a serving platter. Serve hot!

Nutrition: Calories: 149 , Carbs: 10g , Fat: 10g , Protein: 8g

Drinks

Warm Spiced Lemon Drink

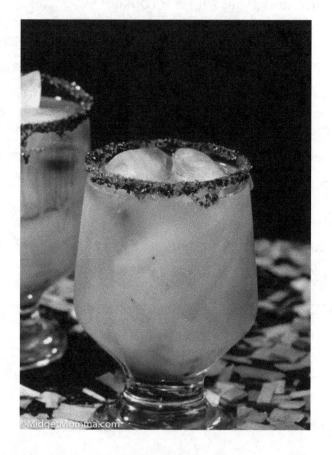

Preparation Time: 10 minutes

Cooking Time: 2 hours

Servings: 12

Ingredients:

1 cinnamon stick, about 3 inches long

1/2 teaspoon of whole cloves

2 cups of coconut sugar

4 fluid of ounce pineapple juice

1/2 cup and 2 tablespoons of lemon juice

12 fluid ounce of orange juice

2 1/2 quarts of water

Directions:

Pour water into a 6-quarts slow cooker and stir the sugar and lemon juice properly.

Wrap the cinnamon, the whole cloves in cheesecloth and tie its corners with string.

Immerse this cheesecloth bag in the liquid present in the slow cooker and cover it with the lid.

Then plug in the slow cooker and let it cook on high heat setting for 2 hours or until it is heated thoroughly.

When done, discard the cheesecloth bag and serve the drink hot or cold.

Nutrition: Calories 523 Carbohydrates: 4.6g Protein: 47.9g Fat: 34.8g

Soothing Ginger Tea Drink

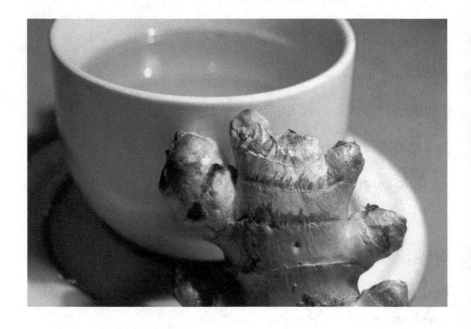

Preparation Time: 5 minutes

Cooking Time: 2 hours 20 minutes

Servings: 8

Ingredients:

1 tablespoon of minced gingerroot

2 tablespoons of honey

15 green tea bags

32 fluid ounce of white grape juice

2 quarts of boiling water

Directions:

Pour water into a 4-quarts slow cooker, immerse tea bags, cover the cooker and let stand for 10 minutes.

After 10 minutes, remove and discard tea bags and stir in remaining ingredients.

Return cover to slow cooker, then plug in and let cook at high heat setting for 2 hours or until heated through.

When done, strain the liquid and serve hot or cold.

Nutrition: Calories 232 Carbs: 7.9g Protein: 15.9g Fat: 15.1g

Nice Spiced Cherry Cider

Preparation Time: 1 hour 5 minutes

Cooking Time: 3 hours

Servings: 16

Ingredients:

2 cinnamon sticks, each about 3 inches long

6-ounce of cherry gelatin

4 quarts of apple cider

Directions:

Using a 6-quarts slow cooker, pour the apple cider and add the cinnamon stick.

Stir, then cover the slow cooker with its lid. Plug in the cooker and let it cook for 3 hours at the high heat setting or until it is heated thoroughly.

Then add and stir the gelatin properly, then continue cooking for another hour.

When done, remove the cinnamon sticks and serve the drink hot or cold.

Nutrition: Calories 78 Carbs: 13.2g Protein: 2.8g Fat: 1.5g

Fragrant Spiced Coffee

Preparation Time: 10 minutes

Cooking Time: 3 hours

Servings: 8

Ingredients:

4 cinnamon sticks, each about 3 inches long

1 1/2 teaspoons of whole cloves

1/3 cup of honey

2-ounce of chocolate syrup

1/2 teaspoon of anise extract

8 cups of brewed coffee

Directions:

Pour the coffee in a 4-quarts slow cooker and pour in the remaining ingredients except for cinnamon and stir properly.

Wrap the whole cloves in cheesecloth and tie its corners with strings.

Immerse this cheesecloth bag in the liquid present in the slow cooker and cover it with the lid.

Then plug in the slow cooker and let it cook on the low heat setting for 3 hours or until heated thoroughly.

When done, discard the cheesecloth bag and serve.

Nutrition: Calories 136 Fat 12.6 g Carbohydrates 4.1 g Sugar 0.5 g Protein 10.3 g Cholesterol 88 mg

Dessert Recipes

Coconut Oil Cookies

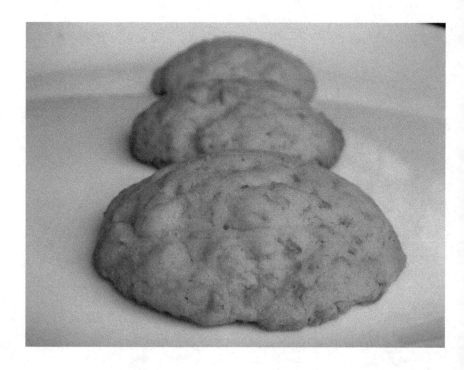

Preparation Time: 10 minutes

Cooking Time: 10 minutes

Servings: 15

Ingredients:

3 1/4 cup oats

1/2 teaspoons salt

2 cups coconut Sugar

1 teaspoon vanilla extract, unsweetened

1/4 cup cocoa powder

1/2 cup liquid Coconut Oil

1/2 cup peanut butter

1/2 cup cashew milk

Directions:

Take a saucepan, place it over medium heat, add all the ingredients except for oats and vanilla, stir until mixed, and then bring the mixture to boil.

Simmer the mixture for 4 minutes, mixing frequently, then remove the pan from heat and stir in vanilla.

Add oats, stir until well mixed and then scoop the mixture on a plate lined with wax paper.

Serve straight away.

Nutrition: Calories: 112 Cal Fat: 6.5 g Carbs: 13 g Protein: 1.4 g Fiber: 0.1 g

Express Coconut Flax Pudding

Preparation Time: 5 minutes

Cooking Time: 15 minutes

Servings: 4

Ingredients:

1 Tbsp coconut oil softened

1 Tbsp coconut cream

2 cups coconut milk canned

3/4 cup ground flax seed

4 Tbsp coconut palm sugar (or to taste)

Directions:

Press SAUTÉ button on your Instant Pot

Add coconut oil, coconut cream, coconut milk, and ground flaxseed.

Stir about 5 - 10 minutes.

Lock lid into place and set on the MANUAL setting for 5 minutes.

When the timer beeps, press "Cancel" and carefully flip the Quick Release valve to let the pressure out.

Add the palm sugar and stir well.

Taste and adjust sugar to taste.

Allow pudding to cool down completely.

Place the pudding in an airtight container and refrigerate for up to 2 weeks.

Nutrition: Calories: 140 Fat: 2g Fiber: 23g Carbs: 22g Protein: 47g

Full-flavored Vanilla Ice Cream

Preparation Time: 5 minutes

Cooking Time: 20 minutes

Servings: 8

Ingredients:

1 1/2 cups canned coconut milk

1 cup coconut whipping cream

1 frozen banana cut into chunks

1 cup vanilla sugar

3 Tbsp apple sauce

2 tsp pure vanilla extract

1 tsp Xanthan gum or agar-agar thickening agent

Directions:

Add all ingredients in a food processor; process until all ingredients combined well.

Place the ice cream mixture in a freezer-safe container with a lid over.

Freeze for at least 4 hours.

Remove frozen mixture to a bowl and beat with a mixer to break up the ice crystals.

Repeat this process 3 to 4 times.

Let the ice cream at room temperature for 15 minutes before serving.

Nutrition: Calories: 342 Fat: 15g Fiber: 11g Carbs: 8g Protein: 10g

Irresistible Peanut Cookies

Preparation Time: 5 minutes

Cooking Time: 25 minutes

Servings: 8

Ingredients:

4 Tbsp all-purpose flour

1 tsp baking soda

pinch of salt

1/3 cup granulated sugar

1/3 cup peanut butter softened

3 Tbsp applesauce

1/2 tsp pure vanilla extract

Directions:

Preheat oven to 350 F.

Combine the flour, baking soda, salt, and sugar in a mixing bowl; stir.

Add all remaining ingredients and stir well to form a dough.

Roll dough into cookie balls/patties.

Arrange your cookies onto greased (with oil or cooking spray) baking sheet.

Bake for about 8 to 10 minutes.

Let excellent for at least 15 minutes before removing from tray.

Remove cookies from the tray and let cool completely.

Place your peanut butter cookies in an airtight container, and keep refrigerated up to 10 days.

Nutrition: Calories: 211 Fat: 18g Fiber: 20g Carbs: 17g Protein: 39g

Conclusion

Congratulations on making it to the end of this cookbook.

Plant-based diets contain a large number of plant-based and antioxidant blends, which appear to reverse psychological deficiencies. A balanced diet not only helps your body lose weight and cope with and prevent some diseases, it also improves your mind. If this is the first plant-based diet you follow, it may happen that you give in, the important thing is to get up and resume your journey. Surrounding yourself with people like you who are trying to follow this lifestyle can be very helpful in motivating you to continue. Remember motivation is the basis of everything, without it nothing is possible. I hope you will be able to reach your goal of a healthy life and weight loss.

Good luck!

CPSIA information can be obtained
at www.ICGtesting.com
Printed in the USA
BVHW052009290421
606130BV00003B/335